Praise for *The Wiser Woman's Guide to Perimenopause and Menopause*:

When you read this book, if you allow the love it is written with to automatically fill your heart, I'm certain you'll wake up to the guidance of your true self far sooner than I did. As a result, you'll have the opportunity to enjoy midlife and beyond in ways you probably haven't even imagined possible. What a gift!

— Dr. Anne Curtis, sexual therapist and permaculture designer, retired family doctor and psychotherapist

This eye-opening, compelling, and transformative book is much more than a guide to relieve perimenopause and menopause symptoms. Tania shines light on the current narrative around women's health and offers a profound and truthful message, allowing women to take back their power and reconnect to their innate wisdom and ability to heal. It's a gorgeous, hopeful, and inspiring read!

— Deborah Binun, BSc, MA, MBACP, psychotherapist and author of *The Missing Peace in Childbirth*

Menopause has come to be viewed as a time in a woman's life when the body is "failing" — a time when women are destined to suffer or medicate their way through. However, there are

wise women who know better and do not fall for this narrative. Women who understand this transition at a much deeper level. Tania is such a woman. She provides us with a loving reminder of the true nature of this journey, one of sovereignty, wisdom, and self-awareness.

You will feel your body relaxing as you read this book. You will feel yourself settling into a deeper level of connection with your being. Allow this, follow this. There is wisdom, beauty, and comfort in these pages.

— Rachel Singleton, transformative coach and creator of *The Beautiful Feeling Podcast*

The Wiser Woman's Guide to Perimenopause and Menopause touched me deeply with its timeless wisdom. This book would have been incredibly supportive when I went through menopause more than a decade ago, yet the gifts that Tania shares are valuable throughout our life-cycles. As I read the book, I felt strongly connected to the eternal Wiser Woman within. I highly recommend this book to women of all ages, especially those wanting a calmer and more soul-led experience of perimenopause and menopause.

— Ellen Friedman, PT, MA, Three Principles practitioner

For all inquiries, including book orders:
thewiserwoman.com/contact

First published in 2022 by:
Flower Cap Press
Israel and USA
ISBN: 978-0-9829759-5-4

THE WISER WOMAN'S GUIDE TO
PERIMENOPAUSE
AND MENOPAUSE

A PATH TO NATURAL SYMPTOM RELIEF AND
AN ENHANCED SENSE OF WELL-BEING

TANIA ELFERSY

The Wiser Woman is within you, and she wants to be found.

TABLE OF CONTENTS

INTRODUCTION   11

CHAPTER 1   CREATION   19

CHAPTER 2   DEPARTURE   33

CHAPTER 3   SHE'S CALLING   51

CHAPTER 4   TRUST   65

CHAPTER 5   PROMISE   85

CHAPTER 6   SOVEREIGNTY   95

CHAPTER 7   LOVE   119

NOTES   133

INTRODUCTION

In 2015, I came across an understanding of innate health that allowed me to heal my perimenopause symptoms simply and naturally. Since then, I have been guiding women to look within and tap into the inherent brilliance of the body so they can heal their perimenopause and menopause symptoms too.

The healing process involves a shifting of awareness, welcoming of insight, and ultimately, a journey of the soul. It's about encouraging each woman to discover The Wiser Woman within and allowing her innate, ancient wisdom to take the lead. When this happens, symptom relief is only the first step. The rewards on this journey are so much greater than that.

If we buy into the story that our crazy hormones are causing us to feel bad, then it seems our path to healing must be complicated and must involve fixing ourselves via pills, patches, creams, and potions — either from natural or more chemically processed ingredients.

In this book, I will explain how it cannot be that our hormones (or any parts of our body) are the source of our discomfort. Despite the dominant narrative that broadly dictates approaches to women's health, our bodies aren't betraying us, and our hormones cannot act outside of a divine intelligence.

However, if you are currently swimming in a soup of symptoms (I do remember how that feels) and have been convinced that your "malfunctioning" body is to blame, I know how unlikely what I'm sharing may seem. Luckily, with years of experience behind me, I can assure you that nobody lives beyond the principles of innate health, and no woman's healing path needs to be complicated — not even yours.

What I describe in this book will hopefully shine a light on a non-physical process that results in changes that can be felt in the physical realm. The English language can be limiting when we describe metaphysical concepts. In addition, words used in the book — *soul, divine intelligence,* and *energetic field,* to name a few — may invoke different things in different people. I encourage you to play with the concepts presented within and switch words in your mind to ones that resonate with you. For example, you may feel more comfortable thinking about God or using the word "source" rather than "divine intelligence" or "The Wiser Woman." Allow yourself to think in terms that you feel connected with.

As you read through the chapters, you may come to understand what is needed in a healing process on an intellectual level, but for a healing process to have an impact, it must be experienced as a shift in consciousness. With this in mind, I encourage you to experiment with the concepts I share whenever you are inspired.

To help this book be a catalyst for a new type of experience, I have kept it short, avoiding long explanations that can send our minds into a swirl as we try to "work things out." Luckily, the understanding that I share is incredibly simple to grasp. Some reject it, believing it is too simple, as if leaps in consciousness occur while we're busy with mind acrobatics. (They don't!) Women have also told me how crazy the ideas that I share seemed to them at first, but then they were inspired to explore more. They relistened to an interview I had given on a podcast or reread some of my blog posts, and with time, they were able to see something new and transformative.

There is no method required to experience symptom relief and transformation, and there is no predictability about how long it will take for change to be felt. Yet, the chances that you will witness major shifts in your life can increase if you are willing to engage and play with what I share in this book.

I hope you'll experience this book in flow. To help that happen, although I have provided detailed notes for further exploration in the back of the book, I did not number the notes within the main text.

Instead, I divided the notes by chapter and explained each one to help you remember what part of the text the note refers to. This will allow you to finish the book without distraction, then explore the notes for further reading. All notes can also be found online at the URL given at the start of the notes section, providing you with quick access to references on the internet.

As always, I welcome all feedback. Feel free to reach out to me via my website at: thewiserwoman.com

CHAPTER 1
CREATION

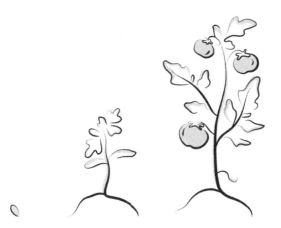

Life is a series of everyday miracles.

My childhood room in our suburban London home was a site of miracles. Miracles of the type we take for granted.

It was a small room with a window that caught the sun. (When the sun shone!) The window was designed with a large windowsill, which was big enough for me to sit on. In early spring, my father would line the windowsill with tiny pots, and in each pot, there was a seedling that had grown from a tomato seed.

A few months on, my father would carry the young plants into the garden. He would set them in the ground and tend to them until late summer when we could eat the fruit they produced.

In today's modern society, perhaps we don't devote enough time to pondering the wonders of plants. However, if, by chance, we remember that a tiny tomato seed is packed with all the knowledge it needs to create a robust tomato plant and a crop of tomatoes, we might feel comfortable calling it a miracle.

Time spent outdoors surrounded by plants and animals can help ignite a sense of wonder if our minds are quiet enough to notice the magnificence of Mother Nature. But rather than marveling at what's going on outside, what if we looked within?

When I grew up, no one spoke of miracles when it came to my body. How about you? And yet, no one had to tell my body how to develop from a baby to a toddler, to a girl, to a teenager, to a woman, and in my case, to a mother of three children. All that knowledge had been stored within and released with perfection — as befitting a miracle!

Before reaching midlife, I was lucky enough to have experienced short periods of awareness of the body as miraculous. Most stunningly, this occurred during my three pregnancies and subsequent births, and while I watched each of my babies thrive from my breastmilk alone.

Perhaps you have experienced miraculous moments from your body, too — times when a logical explanation of what happened in the physical plane could not possibly express the wonder you witnessed.

Maybe, because I had been touched by miracles from within, when I heard the "your hormones are malfunctioning" story while in my mid-40s and experiencing perimenopause symptoms, it challenged me to set off on a path of discovery. Even though I felt like I was falling apart, I started asking questions.

Could it be true that my body, once a site of miracles, had lost its magic?

If I'd felt my body had taken care of me, why would it stop come midlife?

Could my body create something (even symptoms that I experienced as crazy-making) that wasn't sourced from its innate intelligence?

We have moved beyond the times when people in influential places can get away with arguing that women are prone to malfunction during their lifecycles because they are the weaker sex (although some doctors no doubt still hold such beliefs). The only explanation I've heard over the past decade about why women experience so many symptoms come midlife is because "women never used to live much beyond 40!"

If we hear multiple doctors and media personalities sharing such a statement, does that make it true? If it were, doing a little math, we'd find that many children would have grown up without grandmas for millennia, and few would understand how Little Red Riding Hood went to visit hers!

But if it's not true, what might be true instead when it comes to menopause?

In the book of Genesis from the Bible (a text considered to be written over 2,500 years ago), we find the story of Sarah. In chapter 18, verse 11, it is written:

Now Abraham and Sarah were old, coming on in years; Sarah had ceased to have the way of women.

In other words, Sarah had already passed through menopause.

When Sarah overhears a prophecy that she will have a baby, it is written: *And Sarah laughed to herself.*

The text does more than reveal a post-menopausal woman in ancient times (while nothing in the text points to Sarah being unusual in terms of her age). It also reveals a post-menopausal woman with an intimate understanding of what one could expect from a woman at her stage in life — that she couldn't give birth.

The writers of Genesis understand menopause, and the reader is also expected to understand what happens to women post-menopause.

If post-menopausal women didn't walk the earth over two millennia ago, Sarah's story wouldn't be in Genesis.

If we move forward in history to the 2nd century ACE, we find the writings of Galen of Pergamum, a physician who himself lived to be around 80. In his work, which remained central to Western medicine until the 18th century, Galen proposed that when women's periods stopped, they became less feminine and more "manly hearted."

Why would Galen write about menopausal women if they didn't exist in the 2nd century?

Let's move into the 12th century, where we find the work of Hildegard of Bingen. Hildegard was a German Benedictine abbess, mystic, and healer who lived to age 81.

Hildegard wrote about natural history and herbal medicine, giving particular attention to the stages of a woman's lifecycle. On menopause, she wrote in the book *Cause and Cure*: "From the age of fifty or, for some women, sixty, menstruation stops and the womb begins to shrink and contract so she cannot conceive children."

Surely, if very few women lived beyond menopause in the 12th century, Hildegard would have written about this lifecycle change in another way. She appears to point out that fewer women reach menopause in their 60s than in their 50s, not that the experience of menopause is rare itself.

It turns out that it's a misreading of data on life expectancy over the ages that has given rise to the idea that, at one time, women never used to live beyond midlife. It's worth noting that the same data is never misread when it comes to men. I wonder why?

A graph of average life expectancy over the last 500 years, from England, for example, will show a few lines that each run the shape of a hockey stick. The line turns upward in the mid-18th century for the aristocracy and the late 19th century for everyone else.

In 16th century England, the average life expectancy hovered in the late 30s for all classes, but not because women were dropping off at midlife. At this time, society wasn't organized to preserve the health of children. Research suggests that in the 16th century, approximately a quarter of all children died before their first birthday, and almost half died before age 16. These horrific historical trends are what brought the AVERAGE life expectancy to such low numbers.

Societies with a high prevalence of teenage birthing mothers (which puts babies and young mothers at risk), contaminated water supplies, poor nutrition, and child labor have high child mortality rates. Respect for teenage girls, the innocence of childhood, and Mother Earth create harmony in humanity. This, in turn, gives infants and children a better chance in life and increases average life expectancy.

So, if the idea that women never lived beyond menopause is indeed made up, what could cause such an abundance of physical and emotional symptoms and create so much suffering among women come midlife? Could there be a bug in our design? Were our hormone levels never supposed to drop? Could nature itself be getting it wrong?

Without our interference, nature always moves to create balance and harmony. Woodlands, forests, and jungles inherently thrive with harmony between species. We also know that if humans abandon a town or village, nature will take over. Plants push up between concrete slabs, trees grow through houses, animals roam freely, and a whole new ecosystem is created for the simple purpose of allowing nature to thrive in abundance.

Each woman is her own ecosystem — a community of human cells, bacteria, fungi, and other microorganisms that work together to ensure the body functions smoothly. So, why wouldn't our ecosystems be designed to thrive in abundance while in perfect balance? Why would it be part of nature's design that a certain component of the system — our hormones — was programmed to create havoc at midlife? Are we the exception to every other system we see in nature?

No, I don't believe we are. But we have the free will to innocently interfere with what nature seeks to create. **While nature is always seeking balance, we are the variable in creation.**

Our physical, psychological, and spiritual behaviors can either work in coherence with the larger forces of nature or repel them to create a personal field of chaos, which in our bodies, can be impactful indeed.

We are born with an innate program that allows us to thrive at each stage of our lifecycle. Between stages, our transformation is designed to occur smoothly, serving us, our offspring, and the species.

When a woman becomes a mother, for example, a rapid transformation must occur to allow the mother to naturally feel the call to prioritize her baby's needs.

If a lack of early bonding between a mother and her child disturbs this transformation, chaos can unfold in early motherhood and the infant's development.

At midlife, a transformation must also occur to prepare us for our important role as a wiser elder. We are supposed to learn what is needed for a healthy mind, body, and soul so that we can look after our own health and be in a position to guide future generations. However, if, as we've witnessed over decades, there is interference in this transformation whereby change is resisted and medicalized, and lessons are not learned, could the consequences be felt on a multigenerational level?

Why would we want to interfere with the gathering of wisdom as we graduate to the role of elder? If the role of wiser elder is our destiny, shouldn't we be prepared to embrace it and benefit ourselves and humanity along the way?

Chapter 2
DEPARTURE

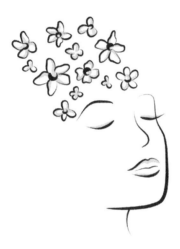

There is less to do than we think.

At the age of 43, my body decided that it was time to wake me up. In my innocence and with my limited awareness of how our bodies communicate with us, I couldn't understand why I felt so bad for so long and was unable to shake it off.

It started with a fever here and there (which, looking back, has always been my body's mode of choice to get me to slow down). Then there were frequent migraines, night sweats, hair loss, mood swings, eczema, and achy breasts.

Stuck in a more natural version of the allopathic model (which promotes a pill or surgical procedure for every ill), I started to look outside of myself for what potion or treatment could make me feel better and more like myself again.

I tried acupuncture, Bach flower remedies, herbal creams and tinctures, and different modes of healing, yet I ended up playing "whack-a-mole" with my symptoms. Although the treatments and remedies offered some relief, I never felt my normal self, and it seemed as if there was always another symptom waiting in the wings to surprise me.

After a few years of running between treatments and with a stock of potions in my bathroom cabinet and tucked into the fridge door, I was lucky enough to come across a webinar on women's health where I heard, "A lot of women in their 40s experience what can be described as PMS on steroids." Instantly, a big penny dropped. PMS on steroids was my monthly experience! This was the first time I heard about perimenopause.

Like many women, I entered my 40s not thinking about The Change — surely, that was at least a decade away! No one had told me that the process of completing my menstrual cycles could take 10 years or more. I'd also never asked.

Just like at the start of menstruation, as our physical development and new hormonal rhythm take time to stabilize, it makes sense that moving on from our reproductive years also happens slowly, over many years.

In 2012, when I started experiencing symptoms, there wasn't much awareness about perimenopause. None of my friends who were in their 40s knew anything about it! Over the previous two decades, medicine had narrowed the definition of menopause to a point in time (one year after a woman's last period). Then they added the term "perimenopause" to cover the years leading up to menopause but forgot to do a good job of updating the public.

I dug out my well-worn 1989 edition of the popular women's health book *Our Bodies, Ourselves* and discovered that the word "perimenopause" doesn't appear. Instead, in the book, menopause is given a broader definition to include the time when women experience menstrual irregularities and other changes years before and after menstruation stops.

In a 1998 edition of the same book, perimenopause is indexed and referred to over two pages. In a 2011 edition, perimenopause is promoted to a chapter title.

I can only speculate why the definition of menopause changed. Perhaps it's connected to the testing for menopause and prescriptions for hormone replacement therapy (HRT). Perhaps it's because, as a society, we found menopause depressing and not something we wanted to experience in our 40s. After all, confining menopause to a 50-something experience fits well with our drive for anti-aging. *Can we please not change for as long as possible, even though change is part of the design?*

Finding out that my symptoms were, in fact, experienced by many women come midlife helped me feel less alone and offered a framework for healing. However, blaming my hormones for how I felt didn't seem like the right path to take.

In 2014, during a glorious family holiday to Thailand, when I wasn't getting my regular acupuncture treatments and mostly forgot to take my Bach remedies and herbal potions, I noticed my symptoms almost disappeared and wondered about that. Do holidays change how our hormones fluctuate? What is the "secret sauce" of holidays that causes many people to have a reduction of all kinds of symptoms — and can we bring that secret sauce back home with us?

When I came back from Thailand, my symptoms started up again. But instead of reaching out to everything I had been doing to bring me relief, it became apparent that it would be a better idea to stop trying to turn down the volume of my symptoms and instead listen to them with curiosity. This was the path I was inspired to take. It was more about being with my body where it was than trying to do something to get somewhere else.

A new perspective started to form, somehow connected to my state of mind while on holiday and how that had impacted my symptoms. I began to see that perhaps my symptoms didn't need to be the focus of my attention, and this allowed me to experience them differently. It didn't make them go away but created a lightness around them. I lost the urgency to fix my symptoms and thus fix myself. I dropped a lot of judgment about what my symptoms meant. Perhaps they were telling me something that, until then, I hadn't been willing to hear.

I rested in openness, ready to see something new without knowing when that would happen. A new sense of trust in my body was emerging. It seemed that I was coming out from a storm — a storm that I had innocently created.

At that time in my life, I was a few years into a self-publishing project, working hard to sell a book that had been born from a labor of love. Before I became a mom a decade prior, I had worked in corporate marketing positions in technology companies. Then I became an at-home mom for six years before being inspired to create a gift book that would support women through the early years of motherhood. I co-authored the book with a good friend who was on a sabbatical year from work and set off alone on a self-publishing journey. The creative process of the book emerged with ease, and the book went on to win four international book awards as well as loving reviews from moms and the media. But as I set myself ambitious sales targets and struggled to get anywhere near them, I felt that I had failed in my little business venture.

In other areas of my life, I had (and still have) a lot to feel grateful for: a loving and supportive husband, three wonderful children, extended family close by, a comfortable home, and my husband's business that had taken off exactly when I stepped down from the role of breadwinner and left the corporate world.

And yet, "I'm not enough" was the thought that often landed in my head as I juggled motherhood and my business. Over the years, I had constructed a belief about myself that I could always set goals and realize them. It was a story that wasn't actually true. I hadn't succeeded in realizing every goal I set, just some of them. But for whatever reason, I believed that story. It felt like my identity. It appeared to me that what was happening in my business was challenging my core.

If only I could sell my books …

I took multiple online business courses and tried to implement what others had found so helpful in their businesses. If only I could implement their ideas better.

And if only I could feel more grateful …

If only I could say my affirmations …

If only I could meditate …

There seemed to be a lot of things that I failed to be doing right. "I'm not enough" felt true and like something I needed to fix. Life felt very serious indeed.

Then, as something began to shift in the months after Thailand, a few acts of synchronicity led to my introduction to The Three Principles of Innate Health. This is an understanding of how Mind, Thought, and Consciousness interplay to create the human experience — in health, business, relationships, and every part of our lives.

The Three Principles were first put into words by the late Sydney Banks, and they reminded me of the work of Eckhart Tolle, Michael A. Singer, and other spiritual teachers — but somehow, they explained life in a simpler way that touched me on a deeper level. Within months, I had an insight into how my relationship with thought was creating my experience.

I saw that if I didn't have, what I called back then "unresolved issues," then I wouldn't have PMS. I saw that I was creating unresolved issues by taking my thinking about any issue seriously. **I saw that taking my thinking seriously was a choice, and if I chose not to take my thinking seriously, life would probably be easier.**

Within that insight, there was no command ("Thou shalt not take thy thinking seriously!") and nothing to do ("Follow these steps to not take your thinking seriously!"). All that had happened was a shift in consciousness, and as a result, I saw that it was possible for me to not take my thinking about anything seriously. It felt like true freedom!

Immediately, I sensed I would no longer have the two weeks of PMS I had been experiencing every month. But to my surprise, within days, all of my emotional and physical symptoms cleared up.

It was shocking, incredible, and humbling. I had been innocently creating stress, which had created an imbalance on the physical level, leading to symptoms. And yet, within me, I had everything I needed to effortlessly heal.

On my journey through perimenopause, I promised myself that if I ever found a way to heal my symptoms, I would share it with others. So, I began to share — timidly and fully aware of how unlikely my experience would sound to many.

Then, nine months on from my insight, there was a crisis in my kids' school with a worrying increase in violent acts and bullying among children. My husband and I decided to lead the move for change. There were parents who joined us and then backed down; parents who supported us but were too afraid to join the meetings; a schoolteacher and the principal who were doing everything in their power to preserve the status quo; and we had to involve the city's educational authority. There were lots of things to think about, lots of frustration and worries about the future, and slowly but surely, my symptoms started to return.

I felt like a fake! I thought I'd healed my symptoms! What was I doing sharing what I had experienced if I was back to night sweats, migraines, skin problems, and extended PMS?

I reached out to a new friend, who, by chance, had an understanding of The Three Principles. We chatted about them over an evening meal. That night, I had another insight: *My default is joy*.

I saw that no matter what, I was OK. I could be angry in a meeting, I could make demands in an email, I could watch other parents and staff act on what made the best sense for them in the moment, and **no matter how frustrating I felt a situation was, I could fall back into lightness because joy was still my default.**

My symptoms disappeared again, and I realized without a doubt how helpful sharing my experience could be.

During the months of back and forth with the school and local authorities, I realized that the fear of what *might be* holds no truth. I learned to listen inward for calm and gentle guidance — nudges about the next steps to take that felt like possibilities instead of constriction. This new awareness allowed us to reach a solution with the school system we could not have imagined when we set out to create change.

I integrated the lessons I had learned and continued to share what I'd seen. Soon, other women began to report how they were experiencing transformation, too, as their symptoms dropped away, their sleep improved, and they reached a greater sense of calm and well-being, all through insight and shifts in awareness.

And at this point, there are probably women reading this thinking: *Well, that's a nice story, but the issues that Tania was dealing with involved her little business and some problems at her kids' school. My issues are far more traumatic and serious. Surely this consciousness stuff is not going to work for me!*

So, here is the good news — the content of our issues does not impact our potential to heal. I've seen this with women I have worked with. In addition, I've heard firsthand accounts from others who were touched by The Three Principles while they had been experiencing distress: a psychiatric patient, a prisoner, a young person caught up in gang culture, and a discharged soldier. In each case, the individual witnessed personal transformation that enabled them to leave past traumas behind and step back into their innate health and well-being.

Before each of my two healing experiences, I had been innocently taking on the role of victim in a circumstance that appeared to be beyond my control. When we drop our victim consciousness — I feel bad because of my business, boss, partner, parent, government, hormones, or whatever one inserts there — we bring responsibility back to us. Then, if we open a level of trust in the body and nature's path, we make space for the energy of healing to work effortlessly.

No matter what we've experienced in the past and what issues we currently face, healing is simpler than we think.

CHAPTER 3
SHE'S CALLING

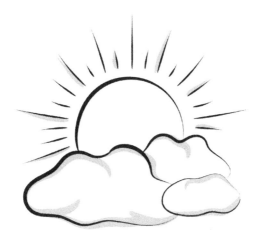

The sun cannot be touched by the weather.

If we believe that healing our symptoms can only happen by fixing our hormones and that menopausal women are peculiar to the modern age, we must conclude that our struggles are with nature's grand plan. Luckily, since these assumptions are not true, the predicament of all women becomes more hopeful.

Within the understanding of The Three Principles, the principle of Mind refers to a divine intelligence behind all things. In my work, when I reference that intelligence as it shows up in a woman's body, I like to call it The Wiser Woman.

Perhaps you would rather call the intelligence God, a divine spirit, or the Universe. It doesn't matter what you choose, as long as you can feel comfortable with the knowledge that it flows through every woman, including you, and we aren't required to control it.

Just as we don't have to tell the heart how to beat, the lungs how to exhale, or our stomach how to digest food, it makes sense that we shouldn't have to tell our endocrine system when to increase or decrease the production of certain hormones. Surely our body, which stores more intelligence than we can yet comprehend, knows what to do and when without us trying to intervene with our modern mindset.

Interestingly, when a woman experiences fluctuations in hormones during pregnancy, we are far less likely to blame her hormones if she experiences symptoms. If a pregnant woman goes to a doctor with swollen legs, exhaustion, and an infection of some sort, the doctor won't declare that it's because of her malfunctioning hormones. A doctor would likely ask the woman about her daily routine, how many hours she's working, perhaps even about her diet. The doctor may then hand out a slip giving her two weeks' leave from work. There is an understanding that pregnancy is a sensitive time in a woman's life, and if she is living a life out of balance, symptoms are more likely to appear.

During pregnancy, the sensitivity of a woman's body makes perfect sense — she needs to protect her baby and herself so they can thrive together, and as a result, so will the species. A body's low tolerance for high stress, long hours of work, and poor nutrition helps enhance this protection. Such a sensitive reaction is not designed to make a pregnant woman's life miserable but to bring her back into balance and in coherence with nature's path. When a woman comes back into balance, she has an easier time in pregnancy, during birth, and postpartum. The sensitivity of her body, created by her fluctuating hormones, is part of the brilliant design!

So, why wouldn't fluctuating hormones at other times in a woman's life — during our teenage years, postpartum, and during perimenopause and menopause — also be part of the body's brilliant design?

During our teenage years, the sensitive time of change encourages us to carve out our path to sovereignty. This is an important step in our maturity that, barring interference, should result in a young adult finding their authority within.

During postpartum, like in pregnancy, the sensitivity a woman experiences is designed to protect her and her child. Unfortunately, at this time in a woman's life, we tend to blame her hormones for any symptoms she might experience (such as postpartum depression). Yet if a postpartum woman lacks love and support from those around her, or if she thinks she should just get back to work or life as usual a few weeks after giving birth because that is what society expects her to do, could these factors not create an imbalance that might be the source of her symptoms? And might the symptoms be a warning sign from the body that the conditions on the ground are not serving her and her baby?

So, what then must be behind the brilliance of design for the sensitivity come midlife? Or, as I like to ask my clients: **What does your body want you to know at this time?**

Most women instinctively know the answer.

Perhaps in our 20s and 30s, our bodies allowed us to get away with a life characterized by high stress, constant fear, a poor diet, or a lifestyle with minimal physical movement; however, in our 40s, the body starts saying *no more!*

The innate intelligence within the body knows what is needed to preserve health as we age into our golden years and starts insisting that a change takes place.

The body can only communicate with us through feelings and symptoms. These are wake-up calls, not signs that our body is betraying us or falling apart. If we choose to suppress the symptoms without becoming curious about what might be creating them, the symptoms can multiply or become louder and more uncomfortable. The body wants us to live and grow older in good health and well-being.

The idea that symptoms are the body malfunctioning rather than an intelligent, loving response to conditions that we, in our innocence, have created goes hand in hand with the medical narrative that disease is inevitable as we age.

Perhaps you have seen graphs showing how rates of chronic disease increase dramatically from midlife on. But do such graphs show us our destiny — or perhaps the destiny of populations living out of balance and in resistance to our innate well-being?

Families and societies thrive when elders are healthy, active, and involved. When our behaviors and lifestyles compromise the chance that we will become such an elder, our body will act on our behalf, and on behalf of humanity, to change our course.

Dan Buettner's study of Blue Zones — areas in the world where average life expectancy is exceptionally high, and rates of chronic disease are exceptionally low — found nine common factors that contribute to longer, healthier, and happier lives. These factors emphasize natural movement, a hopeful mental and spiritual outlook, a natural diet, and connections with family, friends, and community. It's worth noting how many of these factors are absent from much of Western society and how not one relies on FDA or government-driven approval.

Through coaching women in perimenopause and menopause, I have noticed how many, come midlife, start embracing the lifestyles found in the Blue Zones, thanks to their symptoms. Women who were living lives without any form of exercise discover they feel better if they start walking, while other women who used to participate in marathons or triathlons get called to slow down to a form of exercise more in line with natural movement. Many women also notice symptom relief when they clean up their diets; other women are called to make career changes, reducing the hours they work or even shifting to a career they feel more passionate about. And yet, while many of these acts of "doing" can contribute to feeling better, women reach out to me, often having done some or all of the above because they are still experiencing symptoms. As we work together, women discover that the key to transformation lies beyond the physical realm. Healing occurs through a shift in consciousness.

This shift in consciousness involves finding The Wiser Woman within us. Her guidance is available to us at all times, and come perimenopause and menopause, she's bubbling to the surface, calling out to be recognized and encouraging change. She wants to take the lead because her path is that of well-being and the path of least resistance. Through every part of our lifecycle, she is in coherence with nature. At the same time, during our life, we can allow our thinking — the stories and beliefs we hold about ourselves — to create incoherence, which then creates discomfort and symptoms.

Our thinking and moods can change like clouds in the sky. But regardless of the weather, stormy or not, The Wiser Woman is like the sun, present no matter what. She is what you were born with and is the unwavering essence of you — peace, love, and joy.

The suffering that so many women experience from symptoms at midlife comes from the imbalance we create with nature through our lifestyles and a misunderstanding of our responsibilities versus the role of a divine presence.

When we insist that how we feel must be due to our hormones or other chemical imbalances, or indeed any physical circumstance, we ignore the fact that since we are the variable in creation, we must also be the creator of any state that is not in harmony with nature's inherent balance. Yet, when it comes to "fixing" ourselves, we shoulder all the responsibility of the need to do something because we cannot conceive of a greater divine force that we can relax into and partner with to heal.

An awareness of The Wiser Woman in each of us changes this paradigm. Once we see that symptoms and feelings are designed to guide us — a calling from The Wiser Woman — we can stop rushing around looking for the thing (the pill, cream, doctor, or therapist) that will make us feel better and instead, slow down, learn what the body wants us to know, and allow healing to naturally evolve.

When we understand the nature of thought and its role in creating our discomfort, we can change our relationship to thought and spend more time in a higher state of consciousness being led by The Wiser Woman (or divine Mind).

As we examine more about the nature of thought in the next chapter, it's comforting to remember that the divine presence running through us means that we are taken care of. We always have been and always will be, no matter what.

CHAPTER 4
TRUST

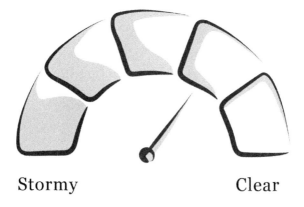

Stormy   Clear

Our feelings are divine guides.

Let's play a mind game.
Imagine you're sitting in a circle of 10 women.

I bring in a chocolate cake and place it on a table in the center of the circle.

The thought "there's chocolate cake" must start as neutral, without any positive or negative charge.

However, as I cut the cake into 10 pieces and start handing it out, there could be 10 different experiences of the same cake, all being created at the same time — 10 separate realities.

Perhaps some of these realities would take on these flavors of feeling:

Calm: I fancy or don't fancy cake. (Here, there is an absence of a personal story interacting with the idea of cake.)

Guilty: I want some cake, but I really shouldn't. How many calories have I already eaten today?

Needy: I've had such a hard day. I deserve a big piece of that cake!

Superior: It's probably not worth the calories. I bet that cake won't taste as good as mine. She probably uses crappy cocoa.

Inferior: Why do my cakes never turn out so good?

Health stressed: I wonder if she uses organic ingredients. There'll be aluminum in the baking powder if she doesn't!

Worried: What if I take a slice and don't like it? Will the host notice and be offended?

Irritated: Why is she offering us cake? Couldn't she bring out some fruit instead?

Anxious insomniac: What's the time, and how much caffeine is in cocoa? I bet if I eat cake now, I won't be able to sleep tonight.

In love: Life is amazing, and how wonderful that we get to eat cake!

Just as each woman in the circle can experience a different feeling, each of us could also experience such feelings while contemplating chocolate cake on different days. Isn't it interesting how that works?

So, what if we replace the chocolate cake with a boss, family member, politician, or slow cashier at the supermarket? Have you noticed how different people experience these things differently? And can our experience of them change without the people themselves actually changing?

When my kids were young, they loved to play a made-up game that involved high-pitched voices. There were days when their playful squeals appeared cute and days when I had to beg my kids to move to another room because the noise felt unbearable. As I experienced this time after time, it became clear to me that if I was in a light, easygoing mood, the noise could pass me by, but if I was in a low mood, chances were I'd have a much more uncomfortable experience of my children playing their game.

So, does that mean that I should have tried to be in a light, easygoing mood all the time?

If we feel calm, we'll have a better experience of most things, but thinking that we must achieve this state of mind to be happy can end up making us unhappy. We're human. Our feelings are unpredictable and fluctuate. Getting serious about being happy can create daily thought storms about what we *should* be doing to have a more pleasant time in life. And if we don't feel happy, we can have a thought storm about why and how we're failing to do what we should be doing!

However, once we are aware that uncomfortable feelings cannot arise from anyone or anything around us but instead come from our state of mind in the moment (which is fluid and always changing without us pulling imaginary control levers to make things a certain way), then shifting to a lighter state of mind occurs effortlessly. No "doing" is required when a shift in awareness is what's at play.

If I am caught up in insecure thinking, pretty much anything, even chocolate cake, can appear to make me feel agitated. As soon as I remember that it's my thinking in that moment that is making me feel that way, space is created between the circumstance and my thinking. In that space, a new, lighter feeling can emerge.

Despite many of us believing that an uncomfortable feeling means something negative is out there, it actually only means that our state of mind *at that specific time* is stuck in a low mode of thinking. The feeling is like a barometer reading, showing us if our thinking is stormy or calm.

When we have an uncomfortable feeling, it is telling us what's true about our thinking in the moment, not the actual circumstance. If we then tune in to a story about how bad it is that we have an uncomfortable feeling, it will be as useful as getting angry at a barometer for showing us there's stormy weather. Of course, if we do that, the stormy weather won't change, and we'll start to feel even worse!

Uncomfortable feelings act like warning signs. You're on an imaginary train to fear/frustration/ disappointment, but you can get off at any time by remembering how your experience in each moment is created.

As soon as we see that we have free will to *not* take any thinking seriously, a choice about how we'd like to feel in each moment becomes available to us. Seeing that choice is all it takes to gently get off the train that is going somewhere we'd probably rather not go. What a relief!

People engage in all kinds of behaviors because they want to feel different. But we can feel different without needing to do or take something when our consciousness shifts. As this happens, we see through the outside-in illusion. Nothing out there could possibly make me feel anything. **A different experience of everything is always available.**

I often recommend to clients that they play with the ideas presented here. Perhaps at first, not with the big issues in their lives where there is a heavy personal story creating interference, but rather with the little things, like noticing how our experience of what we are dealing with at any moment can shift as our thoughts about it effortlessly change. We can notice how this happens, for example, when we find ourselves stuck in traffic, or we start writing an email that we've put off for a long time, or even while washing the dishes.

By noticing how change can happen without effort, we deepen our understanding of how the human experience is created from moment to moment. This, in turn, opens us up to the possibilities of more meaningful transformation in all areas of our lives — even where there is a big personal story at play.

The more we notice, the more experiences we get to "bank," as I like to say! Then, when we find ourselves in the very human condition of a low mood and start convincing ourselves that this situation is different, and it must be that person or thing out there that is making us feel uncomfortable (rather than our *thinking* about whatever is out there), an experience that we consciously banked may spring to mind. This will help remind us that even if right now we can't see the illusion of what is playing out, the possibility that we'll see it remains open to us.

The more experiences we consciously bank, the deeper our understanding of the human mind and spirit becomes. Additionally, our bounce-back rate from a stressed or fearful state of mind to our default peace of mind will be quicker. And when we are in our default peace of mind, we just have a nicer time, no matter what we're doing!

I want to draw on a few examples from my life to shine a light on the interplay of Mind, Thought, and Consciousness. The examples show what happens when separate realities around approaches to midlife emerge and interact. It is worth remembering that a meeting of separate realities happens in every encounter we have with another person, whether they're a loved one or a stranger.

As I write this book, I am aware that it may be met with all kinds of reactions. From the time I first started sharing my ideas about perimenopause and menopause in 2015, women have been keen to offer their feedback on my work. I am sure that for some women, my work resonates with nothing in their energetic field, and I don't expect to hear from them. They don't have any thinking about what I share and so have a neutral experience of it — just as I would, for example, have a neutral experience of someone discussing the advantages of the different tires used on mountain bikes. The types of women

I hear from feel a charge in their thinking about my work — whether that charge is negative or positive. Women have reached out to let me know that they either love or are deeply offended by what I share.

Just as with the chocolate cake, no woman's reaction to my work comes from the words I write or speak; it comes from their thinking about them. And at the same time, if someone reaches out to me and attacks my work, that person can't make me feel bad — but I can certainly have some thinking about their reaction, which, should I get serious about it, could ruin my day.

Several years ago, I was invited to give a talk on perimenopause and menopause to a group of women. A psychotherapist in the audience took offense to what I was saying about what can cause and heal our symptoms. She interrupted me many times, throwing out all kinds of complicated jargon from her profession in an attempt to back her claim that I was wrong. It became quite difficult for me to continue my talk with ease. At the end of the talk, someone else ran up to me and told me that I clearly shouldn't be saying what I was saying because I wasn't a doctor.

When I started out with this work, I did fear that people might not be willing to hear what I had to share because I'm not a medical professional. But with time, I saw that women who were open to a more holistic approach to health found what I was sharing to be transformative. I also saw that no medical professional I encountered was sharing a similar personal journey of natural healing and that I couldn't get qualified from any institution to share my healing experience with more authority because nothing like it existed.

Nonetheless, when I was faced with what happened during the talk, it obviously resonated with something in my energetic field. I felt horrible and feared that the event had been a disaster. I could barely hear the other women who approached me afterward to tell me how much they had enjoyed it. I went home deflated.

By the next day, my mind had settled, and I wondered how bad the talk had really been. Then I received messages from a few more women who were at the event. They shared how my talk had impacted them and given them a wonderful new perspective on midlife change. It wasn't that these women were more convincing in their reactions than the angry women, but it helped me see that it wasn't the talk that had created the different reactions. Women had arrived at the event with different energies, personal beliefs, and states of mind. And that is what created the different experiences.

On another level, the reactions from the women in the group mirrored what we can see happen in our minds. Insecure thinking can often appear like a marching band (or a defensive psychotherapist). Fresh thinking, which can help us have a more pleasant experience of anything we face, often arrives like a whisper (like the women who were touched by my talk and shared their experiences gently with me, one-on-one, as opposed to making a scene in front of a crowd). When we give attention to insecure thinking, we notice the feelings it brings — agitation, constriction, and urgency. On the other hand, when we notice fresh thinking, it appears light, open, and full of possibilities.

The feeling created by our thinking in the moment can guide us to whether there is truth in the thought we are entertaining or not. I have learned that when I feel agitated, contracted, fearful, or frustrated, there's no truth for me in the thoughts that are creating such feelings. However, if I notice a thought that brings with it feelings of calm, openness, potential, or curiosity, maybe I can look there for inspiration and my truth.

Sydney Banks would often encourage people to *search for the feeling*. That doesn't mean we need to go on arduous searches to feel good! Rather, when we become aware of our internal barometer readings — or, as I like to describe it, the divine guidance offered to us through feelings — we'll be called more to hang out in calm feelings because they're more pleasant, and we'll see the truth held within them.

About a year after that talk, one of my blog posts was promoted in a very large, engaged Facebook group of left-leaning, feminist women, mostly in their 40s and 50s. The post challenged the estrogen theory — that we need the very hormone our body is naturally depleting to overcome perimenopause and menopause symptoms. An angry discussion immediately erupted. I was called all kinds of names and even labeled "dangerous." A doctor was so outraged by my lack of credentials that she told me to Google the Dunning-Kruger Effect ... which I did.

The Dunning-Kruger Effect: a cognitive bias in which people wrongly overestimate their knowledge or ability in a specific area. This tends to occur because a lack of self-awareness prevents them from accurately assessing their own skills. (From *Psychology Today*)

Nice!

With so much criticism from the group coming in at a personal level, very few women dared to publicly show an appreciation for my perspective, yet women were signing up for my mailing list and reaching out via email to find out more. The online discussion became so ferocious that the moderators decided to take down the blog post and all the comments. They apologized to the group that they had decided to share such "offensive" content.

Although I didn't exactly have a warm, fuzzy feeling from the personal attacks, I was reeling from being censored. I had no clue what to do. I just knew I needed to wait.

For the next three nights, I woke up at about 3 a.m. with night sweats, but unlike the time when I was dealing with the problems at my kids' school, this time, I didn't panic about the return of a symptom. I knew the night sweats were a sign that I was caught up in my thinking. And I knew that with time, they would pass. That made it much easier to lie awake in the middle of the night. I didn't have a personal story attached to what was playing out. Within days, fresh thinking emerged about the situation. I sent off an email to the group's lead moderator, returned to my work with renewed energy, and carried on with my life. My night sweats went away. The whole saga was another experience to bank!

Every so often, one of my blog posts creates a flurry of love or hate expressed in comments or emails to me, and I've learned there is nothing for me to do but welcome it all. Then a few months ago, a woman wrote me a detailed email quoting my work and explaining how outrageous it was. Feelings of discomfort fluttered through me until I remembered once again what we can so easily forget: how her experience and my experience are created. I didn't need to do anything to change my feelings of discomfort since awareness would take care of that. Then on the same day, the universe was very generous! That evening on a webinar, another woman quoted the very same passage from my work and shared how, when she had encountered those words during the week, she had slipped into days of peace and calm.

Just as women can have different experiences of my work, I can always have a different experience regarding any reaction to my work or to anything or anyone I encounter.

And the same must be true for everyone. Even during the most seemingly challenging experiences we may face, there is always a different experience to be had. Yes, even with the most challenging ones — because our mind knows no limits when it comes to attaching a story to circumstance.

When we are faced with an issue that we consider challenging and we feel uncomfortable, we don't have to work out what the different experiences available to us might be. It's enough to become aware that such a potential exists. With time, our trust that this is indeed true grows, and as a result, even with the inevitable ups and downs of the human experience, life becomes gentler.

CHAPTER 5
PROMISE

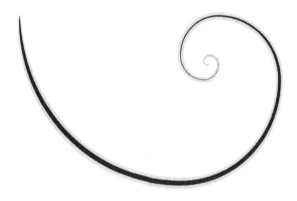

We live in a world of infinite possibilities.

*K*onenki is the Japanese word closest to what we call menopause. It means: *Ko* — renewal and regeneration; *nen* — year or years; *ki* — a season or energy.

Japanese women understand that *konenki* takes place between the ages of 40 and 60. In general, their expectations and experiences of *konenki* differ from and are gentler than Western women's expectations and experiences of menopause.

Research across cultures and even between rural and urban settings has shown how different societies construct menopause. Terms used to describe midlife change, the cultural expectations of women pre- and post-menopause, the dominance of an anti-aging narrative, and the presence or absence of respect for elders may all impact how a woman approaches and journeys through The Change.

There is no universal experience of midlife change across all cultures and settings beyond that at some point, in all women, menstruation stops. This is good news since it further points to the fact that our journeys through perimenopause and menopause can be transformed by seeing something beyond the common beliefs held by the societies we live in.

In English, the terms we often associate with midlife change invoke nothing close to a season of renewal or an upgrade to a wiser elder. As if there weren't enough negative stories associated with perimenopause and menopause, or being "a woman of a certain age," we also have the cultural construct of The Midlife Crisis — a term first promoted in the Freudian psychoanalytical world, which, as it became more broadly referenced, evolved into quite the self-fulfilling prophecy.

A misunderstanding of the nature of the human experience (through confusion around the significance of thoughts and feelings) and/or a misunderstanding of the needs of the human spirit lie at the root of the construct of personal crisis, both at midlife and other times.

Feeling connection, passion, joy, and love are a primal part of a healthy human spirit. When we live without these sensations, over time, our bodies will start creating discomfort, just as if we are deprived of vitamins, minerals, sleep, sunlight, and movement. Come midlife, if our spirit lacks fuel to keep its fire burning beyond a flickering light, the wake-up calls will get stronger. As always, the body knows when change is required to preserve our health in the long run.

When a woman experiences wake-up calls and can't decipher them, perhaps she will try to light her spirit with reactive behaviors that will only bring temporary relief. Or she might light fireworks instead that create disruption beyond her personal life because society has already justified "the midlife crisis."

Luckily, many women I've spoken to over the years have deciphered their own wake-up calls and felt the need to tend to their spirit come midlife — even if they were unaware that this was a divine nudge. Women have been called to follow their desire to paint, write, sing, dance, spend more time in nature, or pursue some other pastime for the sole purpose of feeling connected to their true selves once more.

Others have felt stuck, wishing for change and more time to pursue a passion that is softly calling them. When we feel stuck, we perceive that we are caught between options that seem limited, fixed, and offer unfavorable outcomes.

"I would like more time for myself!" a woman may feel with clarity. "But if I take time for myself, my family or career will suffer. So, I guess I must continue as I am because anything else is impossible."

In 2018, I started my own experiment to discover if, when I found myself feeling restricted by a lack of options, it was actually true. Or in other words, whether I could predict with certainty that the options that I perceived were available to me were indeed the *only* ones available.

I discovered that whenever I felt stuck with a lack of options but then opened myself up to infinite possibilities, more options appeared.

I cannot possibly explain with confidence how that works. I just know it does. I encourage you to doubt me and even if you think my experiment sounds crazy, try it for yourself.

When I encourage my clients to be open to other possibilities when they feel stuck, they are often very pleasantly surprised. Their impossible scenarios — "I can never find time to rest!" "They'll never agree to flexible working hours at my job!" "My kids' father will never agree to that!"— begin to transform and turn out to be not so impossible after all.

Sometimes, we don't even have to play with the concept of infinite possibilities. Surprising developments can occur through understanding more about the nature of thought, which then changes our relationship to the stories we've perceived to be true. When we realize that the stories might not be as fixed as we assumed, we open ourselves up for unpredictable, more favorable outcomes.

It's almost as if during a process of lightening our relationship with thought and feeling, we remove filters from our brain, and our awareness broadens to encompass pathways we couldn't conceive of previously. In short, it's a shift from fear to love, possibility, and clarity. And once you've experienced it, you'll realize you have nothing to lose from playing in the more expansive realms of hope and opportunity again and again.

CHAPTER 6
SOVEREIGNTY

You are sovereign.

Should I start HRT?

Should I switch to bioidentical HRT?

Should I stop my anti-anxiety meds?

Should I undergo that surgical procedure?

These are the sorts of questions women often ask me.

Since I am not a medical professional, I never give advice on medicines and medical procedures. Instead, I help women resolve their questions by encouraging them to reconnect with the brilliance of their bodies and their own authority.

Sometimes medication can be helpful as a first-aid tool to turn down the volume of symptoms when a woman feels her suffering is too great. It isn't always necessary when a more holistic approach to healing is undertaken. But there are cases when it appears as a lifeline, helping a woman navigate to a place where she can understand something new about what is needed to heal.

Just as in creation, we are the variable in healing. We can allow it to progress simply, or we can create interference in nature's path — not because we intend to but because we innocently hold on to a misunderstanding of our innate design.

With the exception of trauma medicine, where a doctor may have to perform miraculous tasks to bring the body back to a state where it can heal, most healing processes require us to get out of the way to allow the body to intelligently bring us back to balance.

With a simple wound, we are required to keep it clean and not pick at it. The body knows how to do the rest.

If we have fallen off the path of good health (rather than crashed), could it be that our role in healing is the same? Keep your body, mind, and soul clean and don't pick at them!

If a woman is experiencing suffering but is yet unaware that she can embrace a relaxed, loving role in the healing process, any medicine she may have started taking as a first-aid measure has the potential to become a lifestyle. In the case of HRT, the lifestyle normally comes with a time limit.

These days, most women who are prescribed HRT during natural menopause will be advised not to take it for longer than seven years because of the increased risk of side effects associated with prolonged use. Many women have reported to me in desperation how all their symptoms came back once they had to stop HRT. No one told them that could happen. They thought HRT had healed their symptoms, but HRT only suppressed them by manipulating the lifecycle. It's a form of medical trickery — now you see a sensitive time of change designed to shape your evolution into a wiser elder, and now you don't.

But I wonder, who's tricking who?

The medicalization of menopause began early last century. It was founded on false beliefs about women's health and expanded through the absence of solid science that would have refuted many of the exaggerated and even fraudulent medical claims made about menopause "cures."

An examination of how medicines were marketed and distributed — and only as an afterthought, thoroughly tested — shows how profits were placed before women's health for decades.

The hormone replacement industry mirrors what has happened in many pharmaceutical segments. And yet, for the machine to keep turning — offering up grandiose promises, downplaying clinical trial results that debunk those promises, then coming back with new, unproven promises — we have to agree to be partners.

For too long, we have thought nothing of handing over our bodies and sovereignty to "the science." But so often, with time, it has been shown that the science is not as health-promoting as we were initially told. Sometimes, it can take decades to reveal the risks associated with approved medical treatments. It is simpler to blame a new health condition on a novel disease, genetics, or even aging than to go back and discover that a negative outcome might be strongly correlated to giving women a certain medicine or treatment.

I will briefly review what is, unfortunately, a scandal-filled history of hormone replacement therapies. We could find similar scandals surrounding medical interventions used during pregnancy and birth (which impacted both mother and infant) and even medical interventions given to children. It isn't easy to accept how the medical system we've placed our trust in has so often given poorly tested medical preparations to *healthy individuals* without disclosing the potential risks and upholding the precautionary principle of medicine — *first, do no harm.*

If you are currently taking HRT or have taken it in the past, please rest assured that every woman's body and experience of midlife change is different, and of course, not every woman who has taken HRT has had a negative side effect. I share what I do because knowledge is power and because I believe it is important to break down the myths about midlife women's health that keep us disempowered.

If you started HRT, it must have appeared the most convincing path to take at the time. If another path seemed more convincing, you would have taken that one. You made the best choices you could with what made sense to you along your journey. That's all we can ever do, each and every one of us!

If I had reached the understanding about health that I have today before I interacted with the medical world at different times in my life, I imagine I would have made very different choices. But is it helpful, loving, or compassionate for me to worry about that now? Judging our past choices is a mind game we have learned to play. In it, we try to convince ourselves that our future lives would look better if we had made a different choice in the past. Isn't that fascinating? Especially considering that the world we live in holds infinite possibilities!

Luckily, no matter where you are in terms of perimenopause and menopause, and no matter what you have chosen to do to help you along your way, **your body remains wise, and your ability to access your innate health and well-being remains intact.**

∞

Before the FDA approved estrogen therapy for menopausal symptoms in 1942, women were offered pills or injections made from animal ovaries to calm their menopause symptoms — because obviously, if a woman's ovaries had stopped working like those of a younger woman, she must need an ovary boost!

The popularity of estrogen therapy started to soar in the 1960s, propelled by the highly influential book *Feminine Forever.* The book was written by a New York gynecologist, Robert A. Wilson, MD, and promoted with funds funneled from Wyeth, the manufacturer of the best-selling estrogen therapy of the time, Premarin.

The book was packed full of myths that would flavor menopause discourse for decades. In it, Wilson described menopausal women as "living decay" and menopause as "a hormone deficiency disease."

He argued that estrogen therapy would "save women from witnessing the death of their womanhood."

Wilson also posited that a WONDER PILL (containing estrogen extracted from **pregnant mar**es' ur**ine**) would cure over 30 menopause symptoms and disorders, reduce the chance of heart disease, stroke, and cancer, PLUS allow women to remain "attractive in tennis shorts or sleeveless dresses." What could possibly be bad?

Despite the complete absence of large, randomized control studies to back up Wilson's claims, he suggested, as was common at the time, that women continue estrogen therapy for life.

Right from the earliest days of estrogen therapy, some doctors were alarmed by the idea that healthy women were going to be increasingly treated with supplemental hormones. Doctors were concerned that since excess estrogen could act as a carcinogen, the risks might outweigh any benefits offered to women going through natural menopause. In 1939, *The Journal of the American Medical Association* (JAMA) even published an editorial entitled "Estrogen Therapy — A Warning."

That warning and others were ignored until 1975, when two important studies were published in *The New England Journal of Medicine* (NEJM). The studies concluded that among women who took menopausal estrogen, the risk of developing endometrial cancer (which arises from the lining of the uterus) was up to five times higher than rates seen in women who didn't take supplemental estrogen and 14 times higher if women took estrogen for more than seven years.

By 1978, the FDA mandated that all estrogen products contain a warning message that estrogen had been proven effective only for hot flashes and vaginal dryness and that estrogen therapy carried risks of cancer and blood clots.

Instead of re-examining the wisdom of boosting a woman's estrogen at a time when her body is naturally depleting it (not to mention, perhaps, the unthinkable — appreciating the innate wisdom of women's bodies!), the pharmaceutical companies, which had already enjoyed tremendous revenues from hormone therapies, decided that a woman's body was the problem because it didn't know how to protect itself from additional estrogen. The solution? Add progesterone to the mix. So progestin, synthetic progesterone, was added to hormone therapies (to protect the uterus), and a combined therapy (which became known as HRT) was offered to women instead.

To overcome "all that bad press" that estrogen increased the risk of cancer, the makers of HRT switched the tone of their marketing to promote the idea that HRT not only offered relief for menopause symptoms but also reduced the risk of osteoporosis and heart disease.

With regard to the osteoporosis claim, studies have shown that estrogen can make a woman's bones denser. However, denser bones do not necessarily equal stronger bones. With prolonged estrogen use, bones are more likely to become dense like glass, making them easy to shatter in the case of a fall. Furthermore, if a woman in her 50s takes estrogen, then stops after seven years (as is common practice), bone density reverses to the levels of pre-estrogen supplementation, meaning that HRT taken during the menopausal years cannot be expected to have a positive impact on bone health later in life.

The belief that HRT could reduce the risk of heart disease had only ever relied on evidence from the results of small-scale trials. The FDA never approved using HRT for this purpose. But it wasn't until the

1990s that the industry got around to commencing the first large-scale clinical trials specifically designed to evaluate the effect of hormone therapy on coronary heart disease (CHD) and women's long-term health. Then, both the Heart and Estrogen/Progestin Replacement Study (HERS), published in 1998, and the Women's Health Initiative (WHI), concluded that HRT did not prevent heart disease. More than that, the Women's Health Initiative was abruptly halted in 2002 because early findings revealed that post-menopausal women taking estrogen and progestin combined hormone therapy had an increased risk of heart disease, breast cancer, stroke, blood clots, and urinary incontinence.

HRT sales went into freefall, and it was time for some crisis management and new messaging. Once the dust settled, the makers of HRT were back with a new spin: We don't need to worry about the results of WHI because the research was "misguided."

The pharmaceutical industry argued that we should discount the results of WHI because the study included the impact of HRT on women who were 10 years and more beyond menopause — as if doctors hadn't just spent decades prescribing HRT to women who were 10 years and more beyond menopause, and that's why those women were included in the study.

None of the dangers posed to older post-menopausal women were relevant to women at midlife, the industry concluded. And with that argument, some prominent doctors returned to convincing menopausal women that leaving menopause "untreated" could increase a woman's risk of heart disease and cancer.

These claims were made even as it became apparent that breast cancer diagnoses had *decreased* dramatically following a drop in the use of HRT due to the publication of the WHI findings. Research around the reduction in the number of breast cancer cases following 2002 led to an estimation that between 1992 and 2002, approximately 200,000 women were diagnosed with breast cancer as a result of taking combined HRT. The courts have also backed up the connection between HRT and breast cancer. Approximately 10,000 women have received or are expected to receive claims of over $1.2 billion after developing breast cancer linked to a single brand of hormone replacement therapy.

We might think that with such a shaky history, medicine would have wanted to be more careful about the unproven promises it attached to hormone therapy. Yet, it seems that because society has been telling us for millennia that women in their natural state are more prone to "malfunction," and there's money to be made from promoting this myth, it's a challenge to see that women's bodies naturally operate in a way that best preserves their health through menopause and beyond.

However, 2017 would prove to be somewhat of a turning point. In that year, *The Journal of The American Medical Association* (JAMA) published the findings of an 18-year clinical trial that investigated the safety of hormone therapies. The trial compared the mortality rates of women who took hormone therapy for a median of six to seven years with women who received a placebo. The research found that women who received hormone therapy were no more or less likely to die of any cause than the women who received a placebo. This led the study's authors to conclude that they "would not support the use of hormone therapy for reducing chronic disease or mortality."

The trial's findings jolted the North American Menopause Society (NAMS) to update their policy statement on hormone therapy and restrict the use of such therapies to the treatment of vasomotor symptoms (night sweats and hot flashes); genitourinary syndromes of menopause (changes to the labia, vagina, urethra, and bladder); and preventing bone loss and fractures. In addition, doctors who had enthusiastically promoted hormone therapy to protect women from disease had to finally stop sharing those fabricated stories.

At least, doctors on one side of the pond.

Since NAMS updated their policy statement in 2017 (which was again updated in 2022, without changing the three categories of symptoms for which NAMS continues to recommend hormone therapy), doctors in the US, who were at the forefront of sharing

112

the myth that hormone therapy prevents disease, changed their story (and updated their websites). But not so in the UK! Even though menopause societies from countries around the world endorsed the NAMS 2017 position statement, the British Menopause Society stood alone in just "supporting" it.

So, in the US, where malpractice claims are significantly higher, doctors are no longer allowed to convince a woman to take hormone therapy for disease prevention, but in the UK, doctors are. To confuse matters even more, pharma interests in the UK have introduced two new strategies for increasing HRT sales: celebrity-backed HRT and a heightened focus on Alzheimer's disease and dementia.

Conveniently, but perhaps not so coincidentally, in 2011 and 2014, the UK government changed the codes used in registering causes of death with regard to dementia and Alzheimer's. This made dementia and Alzheimer's the leading causes of death for women in the UK (while in neighboring European countries where codes had not changed, they are not the leading causes of death).

In May 2022, a celebrity-hosted TV program broadcast on the UK's Channel 4 network claimed that the *long-term use* of HRT would protect a woman's brain and reduce her risk of dementia, Alzheimer's, and other neurodegenerative diseases by up to 80%. The program, which was shamelessly laced with direct pharmaceutical product promotion (despite the strong UK advertising laws that are supposed to prevent such activities), garnered attention from multiple national media outlets before and after its broadcast. The program was so convincing in its claims that it set social media on fire, with women terrified that they were putting their health at risk by *not* taking HRT.

The hysteria around the TV show reached such heights that even the British Menopause Society decided to put out a statement to distance themselves from it. They stated: "HRT should not be initiated for the purpose of reducing the risk of dementia in postmenopausal women and at this time, there is not enough evidence to support prescribing HRT for prevention of dementia."

The messaging around HRT continues to send women on rollercoaster rides. But could bioidentical HRT be any better? A bioidentical HRT product derived from wild yams certainly sounds better than a product containing estrogen derived from horse urine! However, bioidentical HRT is not suitable for everyone. Some women experience undesirable side effects while taking such products, just as some women experience undesirable side effects while taking HRT. Furthermore, bioidentical HRT products vary hugely, and there is scant research on their possible long-term effects on a woman's body.

Using bioidentical HRT may not be as benign as perhaps eating a wild yam (which is packaged by nature), and most importantly, following decades of research by scientists trying to prove otherwise, there is still no evidence that women actually need either form of HRT. It's the myths about women's health — that at a certain time in life, women's bodies start getting the hormonal balance wrong — that fuel both the bioidentical HRT and HRT industries.

As long as societies are structured in ways that don't acknowledge our bodies as inherently wise and, in addition, promote a "fix me quick" mentality, there will be a flow of money invested in doctors, the media, and even celebrities to ensure they are up to date on the current pharma marketing spin and the latest fears of the "malfunctioning" midlife woman. This helps the industry's messaging reach a wider audience and creates a growing base of long-term customers.

Medicine prescribed for long-term use is an attractive business model that not only delivers recurring revenue streams but also has the potential to create multiple *new* revenue streams for the pharmaceutical industry.

Overworked doctors who treat a patient with symptoms rarely take the time to investigate what in the patient's life might be out of balance upstream from the site of the symptoms. But if the original imbalance isn't addressed and instead, symptoms are suppressed, the imbalance can go on to cause new symptoms, and the long-term use of certain medicines can go on to create side effects, all of which may then be treated with additional medications.

At midlife, when so many women start on a path of long-term medication, we have a choice. We can become caught up in a profit-driven medical system — which keeps us dependent on external "fixes" for symptom suppression, yet in the dark about what true risks or benefits may be associated with promise-filled therapies — or we can take an empowering journey back to our innate health to be free.

Even if we are experiencing multiple symptoms, we don't need to be fixed, and we also don't need to go it alone. We need the inspiration and support that will allow us to tune in to what is going on in our body, see how perhaps our soul has drifted from its default healthy path, and accept a loving role in our own healing. Once we take back our authority, we can sit in our sovereignty, wear our crown, and look within for answers. There we'll find the guidance we need to heal and embrace a healthy and joyful life.

Chapter 7
LOVE

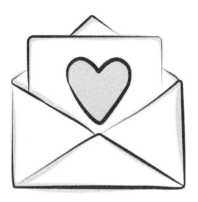

**What if midlife is an invitation to
love yourself deeply?**

I'm writing this book in the summer of 2022. For many of us, the last few years have come with previously unimaginable challenges. While we were never all in the same boat, we all have an innate resilience, which we have leaned into, consciously or not, to keep on sailing.

If I were to list on paper all the events of the last two-and-a-half years that I have wept over, it would certainly appear that this period has been the most challenging of my life. And yet here I am, totally fine, knowing that I was never any less.

It's no longer important what the challenges I faced were. They have all passed. As I view a bigger picture of what played out, I can even see how some of the challenges became gifts. My experience of them, as our experience of anything we encounter, is constantly changing. I cannot force the change, but through an awareness of how experiences are created, I can allow organic transformation to occur with more ease.

As events of the last few years played out, I felt grief, anger, disbelief, frustration, disappointment, and more. There were also moments when something new occurred to me, and I could leap beyond the circumstances. I was inspired to play in new energy realms, with deeper love that I could bathe in and send out beyond my physical boundaries.

"All that is needed," a dear friend liked to remind me, "is to stay in a loving feeling."

And I saw the truth of that. Not through forcing myself into a loving feeling but by falling back into it when I remembered I could — and holding compassion for myself when I couldn't.

A loving feeling is where we came from. It has always been home — our default setting. The feeling creates possibilities, lightness, and well-being in its most expanded and holistic sense. That feeling is the source of transformation to higher states of consciousness.

Five years ago, I started a different version of this book, and it sat one-third written on my computer. I wondered if it would ever be completed. I held the wonder lightly, aware that, in the meantime, my understanding continued to deepen. I was sure I would be called back to the book at the perfect time.

In the spring of this year, I started to play with my vision, quite literally.

Since I believe in the body's innate ability to heal, my slowly deteriorating eyesight perplexed me. I started wearing glasses full-time in my mid-30s and moved to multifocal lenses about 10 years ago. I had the sense that as my numbers edged up each time I bought a new pair of glasses, perhaps I wasn't seeing something about my eyesight.

I had set an intention to see clearly without glasses a while ago, even though I had no idea how that was possible via a natural route. When earlier this year, a good friend told me about a workshop that could improve my eyesight, I was intrigued to find out more, and we decided to go together.

After two days at the workshop, while being without glasses and engaging in different exercises, I definitely felt something had shifted. I also sensed that my eyes were sad to return to my multifocal lenses.

The day after the workshop, I hurried to my local optician and asked for an eye test. The computer gave a reading of the multifocal prescription for the farsightedness of the glasses I was wearing at the time (which wasn't too bad since it turned out I hadn't renewed them in over three years). But the manual eye chart test showed that my eyesight had improved by at least one number for both distant and close activities. I ordered two new pairs of glasses — one for driving and one for reading. When I told the optician I was trying to improve my eyesight naturally, he thought I was mad, even though my performance with the eye chart (when he compared it to the computer readout) had surprised him.

Over the next few months, I tried to find time to do my eye exercises. Although they were clearly helpful, they mostly felt like a chore, which I didn't like. Then, I read about the possibility of spontaneously healing one's eyesight, and I liked that idea much better! It became clear that it would be helpful if I could regularly find time to sit without glasses.

I live a 15-minute drive from the beach. Since becoming a mom, it had seemed (at least to me!) that trips to the beach in the summer should usually include the whole family. However, with our three kids in their mid-to-late teens, it was getting harder to convince them to come along. I realized I could set aside time to go to the beach by myself. I knew the expansive views would be relaxing for my eyes, and I love the beach — I love the sun, lying on the sand, and watching the waves. I always have.

I started going in the mornings. On day two, I noticed how well I could see the detailed patterns on shells, the grains of sand, and the texture of my beach towel, all without glasses. On day three, I took a book with me and realized I could read it on the beach, glasses-free!

Going to the beach became a morning ritual I could manage to fit in up to four times a week. But each day, as I stepped out the door with my beach bag, a dozen reasons sprang to mind why I shouldn't go. It seemed I needed to grant myself special permission again and again.

At night, as I reflected on my day, "I went to the beach" could enter my mind with a sense of fulfillment and gratitude or a tinge of guilt because I was having such a lovely time. That was interesting! Was I allowed to spend so much time at the beach alone?

"You're looking tanned," noted some family members and friends. I explained that I was healing my eyesight at the beach, even though I knew that wasn't the only thing happening. There was also a lot of self-nourishing — grounding in the sand and connecting with the energy of the sun and sea. It was clear that I was calming my soul.

Sometime during the second week, I wondered what else might evolve from my beach time. Then one day, as I lay on the sand, the inspiration for the chapter titles of this book emerged. It became obvious that I could start writing again.

And so, this book was born from my love of the beach, my curiosity around how I could improve my eyesight, my passion for health and healing, and because I allowed myself to go, one step at a time, along a path of bliss that gently called me.

My eyesight has continued to improve, although I don't know when or if I'll be able to set my glasses aside for good. In the meantime, where I can, I take my glasses off and am getting more and more used to being without them. It's a humbling and fascinating journey that, most of all, requires relaxing into where you are and tapping into a state of consciousness that allows seeing to be effortless because, quite simply, "the harder you try, the less you see." It's no surprise that, in essence, this is similar to what I encourage my clients to experience to see something fresh about their journeys toward healing their perimenopause and menopause symptoms.

When we seek personal transformation, it's easy to get caught up in the sense that there must be a lot of "doing" involved. Yet, what if it turns out that experiencing transformation is never more complicated than beholding the beauty and wisdom of nature, embracing its guidance, and falling back into love?

I wonder what the world would look like if we could let nature and love lead us. What everyday miracles might evolve? How much healthier would our lives be?

Over the last few years, I have seen how a loving feeling can heal and transform my being and beyond. I'm grateful for such a valuable lesson that has its roots in connecting to the divine within — the eternal wisdom of The Wiser Woman. She is love on nature's path. She is me, and she is you.

If you would like to continue engaging with the concepts presented in this book in a practical way, I'm delighted to offer you **20% OFF The Wiser Woman Course.**

Through audios, exercises and guided meditations, this three-week online course provides you with a loving and gentle framework to completely transform your experience of midlife change.

Find out how the course can help you reach symptom relief and more:

thewiserwoman.com/the-wiser-woman-course

And enter the discount code **READER20** when prompted at checkout.

NOTES

Access online references with ease! These notes can be found at:

thewiserwoman.com/book-notes

Chapter 1 – CREATION

1. A YouTube video about *'Nightmare' Perimenopause Symptoms*, on the channel **Loose Women**, is an example from the UK of how the life expectancy myth is kept alive. A celebrity (at 1:30) and a well-known doctor and menopause expert (at 9:22) both share the made-up idea that in Victorian times, you'd reach menopause and die. This argument becomes their foundational reasoning for why we need hormone therapies. But if the foundation is faulty, what other "scientific facts" that they share in the interview might also be wrong? As I mention in Chapter 6, in the US, doctors no longer publicly claim that HRT reduces your risk of disease. If you watch the whole interview, you'll see how this is not the case in the UK.

2. For a review of how menopause is referenced throughout history, I recommend the book ***Hot***

Flushes, Cold Science: A History of the Modern Menopause by Louise Foxcroft.

3. For more on the writings of Hildegard of Bingen, see the book *Hildegard of Bingen: Essential Writings and Chants of a Christian Mystic* by Dr. Sheryl A. Kujawa-Holbrook.
   The quote on menopause from *Cause and Cure* can also be found by searching Google Books.

4. Data on average life expectancy in England taken from *A Theory of Medicine Effectiveness, Differential Mortality, Income Inequality and Growth for Pre-Industrial England* by David de la Croix and Alessandro Sommacal, published in *SSRN* (2006).

5. Data on infant and child mortality rates through the ages sourced from *Infant and child death in the human environment of evolutionary adaptation* by Anthony A. Volk and Jeremy A. Atkinson, published in *Evolution and Human Behavior* (2013) and available for viewing in *ResearchGate*.

6. For more information on how infant mortality increases among babies born to young adolescent birthing mothers, see *The impact of young maternal age at birth on neonatal mortality:*

Evidence from 45 low and middle income countries by Sarah Neal, Andrew Amos Channon, and Jesman Chintsanya, published in ***PLOS ONE*** (2018).

7. For a discussion on the wide-ranging consequences of high rates of adolescent birthing mothers in Africa, see ***Teenage pregnancy in Africa: Trend and Determinants in the 21st Century*** by Opeyemi Oluwafunmilayo Odejimi and Denise Bellingham-Young, published in ***ResearchGate*** (2016).

8. A broader discussion on the life expectancy myth can be found in my blog post: ***We are supposed to live this long! Debunking the second biggest myth surrounding peri/menopause.*** thewiserwoman.com/blog

9. For further insight into how we are the variable force in creation, I recommend watching the talk ***Spontaneous Evolution*** by Dr. Bruce Lipton, which can be found on YouTube.

Chapter 2 – DEPARTURE

1. It was during a Hay House webinar that I heard Dr. Christiane Northrup compare the experience of many women in their 40s to "PMS on steroids."

2. The first book I read on The Three Principles that deepened my understanding before my first insight was *The Inside-Out Revolution: The Only Thing You Need to Know to Change Your Life Forever* by Michael Neill. Highly recommended!

3. For further information on the work of Sydney Banks, including videos and a list of his books, which can help you gain a deeper understanding of The Three Principles, visit:
sydbanks.com
sydneybanks.org

4. Many podcasts share The Three Principles understanding. I recommend:
Caffeine for the Soul with Michael Neill (hundreds of short podcasts).
A Little Peace of Mind with Nicola Bird (earlier episodes tend to be longer, later episodes are shorter).

Changeable with Dr. Amy Johnson.

Misunderstandings of the Mind with Jason Shiers.

5. For a fascinating look at how The Three Principles can impact people even after they have experienced trauma and/or a psychiatric diagnosis, I recommend a series of talks with Dr. Bill Pettit, hosted by Elizabeth Lovius, found on the *Real Change Portal* channel on YouTube.

Chapter 3 – SHE'S CALLING

1. Find out more about the lifestyles of people who live in Blue Zones (areas of the world where the average life expectancy is exceptionally high, and rates of chronic disease are exceptionally low) at: bluezones.com

Chapter 5 – PROMISE

1. For more information on how Japanese women experience midlife change, see the book *Encounters with Aging: Mythologies of Menopause in Japan and North America* by Margaret M. Lock.

2. For a fascinating review of the construction of the midlife crisis and lots more, see the book *Life Reimagined: The Science, Art, and Opportunity of Midlife* by Barbara Bradley Hagerty.

3. For a deep dive into the nature of a woman's spirit, I recommend the seminal work *Women Who Run with the Wolves: Myths and Stories of the Wild Woman Archetype* by Clarissa Pinkola Estés.

4. To understand more about the transformations that can occur when we move from fear to love, I highly recommend:

   - The book *Dying to Be Me: My Journey from Cancer, to Near Death, to True Healing* by Anita Moorjani.

   - *The Waking the Wild Show* podcast, hosted by Lian Brook-Tyler, episode 376: *What near death experiences teach us about living more beautiful lives* with Dr. Bruce Greyson.

Chapter 6 – SOVEREIGNTY

1. How safe are FDA-approved drugs? Research from Yale University, published in 2017, found

that nearly one-third of all drugs approved by the FDA have a new safety issue that comes to light in the years post-approval. Read *New safety concerns identified for 1 in 3 FDA-approved drugs*, published in *Yale News*.

2. **Regarding medical preparations given to pregnant women:**

a) Diethylstilbestrol (DES), a synthetic form of estrogen, was prescribed to pregnant women between 1940 and 1971 in the US and until 1978 in Europe to prevent miscarriage, premature labor, and other pregnancy complications. The drug was later found to be ineffective. Research carried out over decades found increased risks of 12 health conditions among daughters of women who received DES while pregnant. These include a twofold higher risk of infertility and a fivefold higher risk of having a preterm delivery. DES-exposed daughters were also found to have an increased risk of some cancers.

To learn more, read *The Long-Term Effects of In Utero Exposures — The DES Story* by Annekathryn Goodman, MD, John Schorge, MD, and Michael

F. Greene, MD, published in *The New England Journal of Medicine* (2011), available for viewing in *ResearchGate*.

b) In the late 1950s and early 1960s, thalidomide was widely prescribed to pregnant women to prevent nausea. It was found to be linked to approximately 10,000 cases of babies born with birth defects. To learn more, read *Thalidomide: The Tragedy of Birth Defects and the Effective Treatment of Disease* by James H. Kim and Anthony R. Scialli, published in *Toxicological Sciences* (2011), available for viewing at: gvsu.edu

c) Have we learned any lessons from history? Consider the present-day case of sodium valproate — a drug given to patients diagnosed with epilepsy, bipolar disorder, or severe migraines.

After **three decades** of public campaigning to bring attention to the harm caused to infants born to mothers who were exposed to sodium valproate, in 2018, the UK Medicines and Healthcare Products Regulatory Agency

(MHRA) issued a statement stating: "Valproate must no longer be prescribed to women or girls of childbearing potential unless they are on the pregnancy prevention programme." Yet in 2022, a **Sunday Times** investigation revealed that doctors were still prescribing the drug to women of childbearing age without disclosing the risks involved. In women who have taken valproate during pregnancy, around 1 in every 10 babies will be born with birth defects, and 3 to 4 in every 10 children will have learning and development problems.

For more details, read:

- *Why is sodium valproate still being prescribed to pregnant women?* This statement was issued by *Leigh Day*, a legal firm representing families bringing medical negligence claims related to problems caused by sodium valproate in pregnancy.

- *Sodium valproate medicines and risks in pregnancy*, an information sheet from *Epilepsy Action*, a UK-based charity.

3. **Putting healthy children at risk in the name of disease prevention.**

a) The legacy of DDT: In the middle of the last century, it was considered beneficial to spray children directly with DDT to supposedly prevent the spread of malaria and other diseases. In 1972, in the US and other parts of the world, the use of DDT was banned because of its toxicity and, in particular, severe neurological disorders that could arise from exposure. The toxicological profile of DDT can be viewed on the website of the *Agency for Toxic Substances and Disease Registry*.

In the YouTube video *Pesticides - DDT - Rachel Carson - Silent Spring*, watch incredible footage of how healthy children and whole neighborhoods were sprayed with DDT and hear the voice of Rachel Carson, author of the book *Silent Spring*, whose research was crucial in halting the use of DDT.

In addition, see how *Like It or Not, DDT Is Good for You*, by Thomas H. Jukes, an article published in *The New York Times* (1971), has an eerie familiarity about it — in the name of "public health," we must keep on doing what we've been doing, no matter what.

b) Have we learned any lessons from history? Consider the present-day case of medical preparations administered to babies to prevent hepatitis B.

Hepatitis B is believed to be caused by a virus transferred between people via blood and other bodily fluids. It is also believed that a mother who carries hepatitis B can pass on the disease to her baby during birth. There is a standard test that medical experts claim can determine if someone is a carrier of hepatitis B, and that test could be given to pregnant women. But in 1991, in the US, it was decided that babies should receive an injection on their first day of life to protect them from hepatitis B. We had better hope that such a product was thoroughly tested before being administered. But was it?

Two such products are currently authorized by the FDA to be given to infants after birth.

Before FDA approval, the makers of one product ran a clinical trial involving **147** healthy infants and children (up to 10 years of age) who were monitored for **5 days** after each dose, while there was **no control group**. Note: We don't know how many infants were included in the trial. See the details of the trial in point 6.1 of the product's package insert at:

fda.gov/media/74274/download

Before FDA approval, the makers of the second product ran clinical trials involving 5,071 healthy adults and children. All subjects were monitored for **4 days** post-administration, while there was **no control group**. Note: As with the first product, we don't know how many infants were included in the trial. See the details of the trial in point 6.1 of the package insert at:

fda.gov/media/119403/download

Two additional "safety studies" (available in *PubMed*) regarding the above-mentioned products were conducted post-marketing, this time with a control group. One study monitored children for 29 days, and the other study for 21 days.

If either of the products increased the risks of any chronic diseases and conditions that would be diagnosed beyond the first month of a child's life, these trials and studies would not have detected such occurrences.

Considering that these products are given to babies on their first day of life, and considering that more than **40%** of US children will be diagnosed with at least one chronic disease or condition before age 18 — a staggering but rarely discussed growing health crisis, detailed in *A national and state profile of leading health problems and health care quality for US children*, published in *Academic Pediatrics* (2011) — why would the scrutiny offered by the FDA be so weak?

4. *Feminine Forever* by Robert A. Wilson is available secondhand if you wish to own an incredible example of the contempt held in the medical world for menopausal women. It's also interesting to read the relatively recent 5-star reviews on Amazon. After all this time, people still believe the fabricated claims in this book!

5. Read *Estrogen Therapy—A Warning*, published in *The Journal of the American Medical Association* (1939).

6. The cancer risks associated with estrogen therapy received public attention when *Editorial: Cancer risk and estrogen use in the menopause*, by K.J. Ryan, was published in *The New England Journal of Medicine* (1975). The article is, as of this writing, behind a paywall but an abstract can be found in *PubMed*.

   In addition, an article (written at the time about the research), *Estrogen Is Linked To Uterine Cancer*, can be found in *The New York Times*.

7. Osteoporosis: Although *The 2022 hormone therapy position statement of The North American Menopause Society* states in its abstract that the therapy "has been shown to prevent bone loss and fracture," when one reads through the osteoporosis section of the document, it also states:

"The BMD [bone mineral density] benefits of preventing bone loss persist as long as therapy is continued but abate rapidly when treatment is discontinued. Within a few months, markers of bone turnover returned to pretreatment values, whereas BMD fell to pretreatment levels within 1 to 2 years of stopping therapy."

Read the full statement on the NAMS website at: menopause.org

8. For an expanded discussion on osteoporosis and HRT, with extra references, read my blog post: ***Osteoporosis, bone health, menopause, HRT, and the confusing messages of medicine***. thewiserwoman.com/blog

9. Read the findings of the ***Heart and Estrogen/ Progestin Replacement Study — HERS***, published in the ***American College of Cardiology*** (1998), which found that HRT offered "no overall cardiovascular benefit" while it "did increase the rate of thromboembolic events and gallbladder disease."

10. Read the principal results from the ***Women's Health Initiative*** randomized controlled trial, ***Risks and benefits of estrogen plus progestin in healthy postmenopausal women***, published in ***The Journal of the American Medical Association*** (2002), available for viewing in ***PubMed***. The trial was halted because "health risks exceeded benefits from use of combined estrogen plus progestin."

11. For a more detailed review of the "changing science" around menopause hormone therapies in the 20th century and up to the publication of the Women's Health Initiative in 2002, I recommend the book ***The Greatest Experiment Ever Performed On Women: Exploding the Estrogen Myth*** by Barbara Seaman.

12. In 2009, **CNN** reported that between 1992 and 2002, approximately 200,000 women were diagnosed with breast cancer as a result of taking combined HRT. In the article ***Study: Hormone therapy caused breast cancer for thousands***, CNN quoted Dr. Rowan T. Chlebowski, a medical oncologist at the Los Angeles Biomedical

Research Institute at Harbor-UCLA Medical
Center in Torrance, who was the lead author
of the research paper *Breast Cancer after Use
of Estrogen plus Progestin in Postmenopausal
Women*, published in *The New England Journal
of Medicine* (2009). The paper concluded that
"the increased risk of breast cancer associated
with estrogen-plus-progestin therapy declined
markedly soon after discontinuation of the
therapy and was unrelated to a change in the
use of mammography. This finding supports
the hypothesis that the recent reduction in
the incidence of breast cancer among women
in certain age groups in the United States is
predominantly related to a decrease in the use of
combined estrogen plus progestin."

13. To read more about the payments made to
women whose breast cancer diagnosis was found
to be connected to a single HRT brand, see
*Prempro Settlements to Result in $1.2B Payments
for Breast Cancer: Report.*
aboutlawsuits.com

14. For an example of the industry pushback to convince women that estrogen therapy prevented chronic disease, read *The Mortality Toll of Estrogen Avoidance: An Analysis of Excess Deaths Among Hysterectomized Women Aged 50 to 59 Years* — research from Yale, published in the *American Journal of Public Health* (2013). The researchers studied women who had **undergone a hysterectomy** but made these general statements in the results and conclusion, respectively: "Over a 10-year span, starting in 2002, a minimum of 18601 [18,601] and as many as 91610 [91,610] postmenopausal women died prematurely because of the avoidance of estrogen therapy (ET)." And "ET in younger postmenopausal women is associated with a decisive reduction in all-cause mortality, but estrogen use in this population is low and continuing to fall." Note how the fact that the study only included women post-hysterectomy (not mentioned in the results or conclusion) was obscured in some media reporting of the research, as if a woman going through natural menopause should be

expected to have the same experience as a woman after a hysterectomy.

A 2013 headline in the *LA Times* warned: *Avoiding estrogen therapy proved deadly for nearly 50,000: study*. That the study was only of women post-hysterectomy appeared in the small print.

A few years later, a 2016 article in *The New York Times* entitled *Rethinking the Use of Hormones to Ease Menopause Symptoms* stated, "In an analysis in 2013 in the *American Journal of Public Health*, Dr. Philip M. Sarrel and his co-authors calculated that, based on reduced death rates among women taking only estrogen in the W.H.I. study, avoiding hormone replacement resulted in the premature deaths of 18,601 to 91,610 women in the decade after the study's release."

15. Read *Menopausal Hormone Therapy and Long-term All-Cause and Cause-Specific Mortality*, the findings of an 18-year clinical trial, published in *The Journal of the American Medical Association* (2017), which jolted the North American Menopause Society to update their position statement on hormone therapies.

16. Read *The 2017 hormone therapy position statement of The North American Menopause Society* at: menopause.org

17. Read *The 2022 hormone therapy position statement of The North American Menopause Society* at: menopause.org

18. Compare to the North American Menopause Society *Global Consensus Statement on Menopausal Hormone Therapy* from 2013 (while noting their position on coronary heart disease and all-cause mortality), at:
menopause.org

19. Compare to the *Joint position statement by the British Menopause Society, Royal College of Obstetricians and Gynaecologists and Society for Endocrinology on best practice recommendations for the care of women experiencing the menopause* from 2022 (while noting their position on atherosclerosis progression, coronary heart disease, cardiovascular health, and all-cause mortality), at:
thebms.org.uk

20. Regarding the changes to the codes used in the UK when registering causes of death related to dementia and Alzheimer's, read *Leading causes of death, UK: 2001 to 2018*, published by the *Office for National Statistics* at:
ons.gov.uk

21. For an in-depth review of tactics recently used in the UK to increase HRT sales, including the highly impactful celebrity-hosted TV program broadcast in May 2022, read my blog post: *Calm after the storm: perimenopause, menopause, the brain, HRT, dementia, and Alzheimer's.*
thewiserwoman.com/blog

22. Read the *BMS [British Menopause Society] comment on [the] Channel 4 programme*, wherein the organization distances itself from promoting the use of HRT to prevent dementia and Alzheimer's, at:
thebms.org.uk

23. For an example of how one leading advocate of bioidentical hormone therapy has relied on the same theories about midlife women's health as some promoters of conventional hormone

therapy, read a testimony given by T.S. Wiley at a Special Committee on Aging in the United States Senate in 2007. The testimony states: "Since we've established that menopausal symptoms are the same symptoms 'old' people experience, then, *menopause must really equal sick*, and since all those outcomes above of 'sick' can be life-threatening, menopause, itself, must really be *life-threatening*."

You might find the statements on page 4 of the testimony to be equally interesting! The testimony can be found at:

aging.senate.gov

24. Is it time to take a fresh look at our relationship with the medical system, including the use of prescription drugs? Watch the presentation *Evidence-Based Medicine Has Been Hijacked* by Dr. Aseem Malhotra on YouTube.

And listen to *The Peter Attia Drive Podcast*, episode 209, an interview with Marty Makary, MD, MPH. Jump straight to 32:30 to learn about the studies showing the ubiquitous nature of medical mistakes that lead to patient death and injury.

Chapter 7 – LOVE

1. I attended a Natural Vision Improvement workshop run by Meir Schneider, PhD, LMT, who healed his eyesight at age 17 after having been blind from birth. Find out about his work at: self-healing.org

2. I found out about the possibility of spontaneously healing one's vision from Dr. Jacob Israel Lieberman. Find out about his work at: jacobliberman.org

   The quote "the harder you try, the less you see" is from Dr. Lieberman's book *Take Off Your Glasses and See: A Mind/Body Approach to Expanding Your Eyesight and Insight*.

Printed in Great Britain
by Amazon

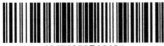

40475950R00091